Let's learn about nursing today!

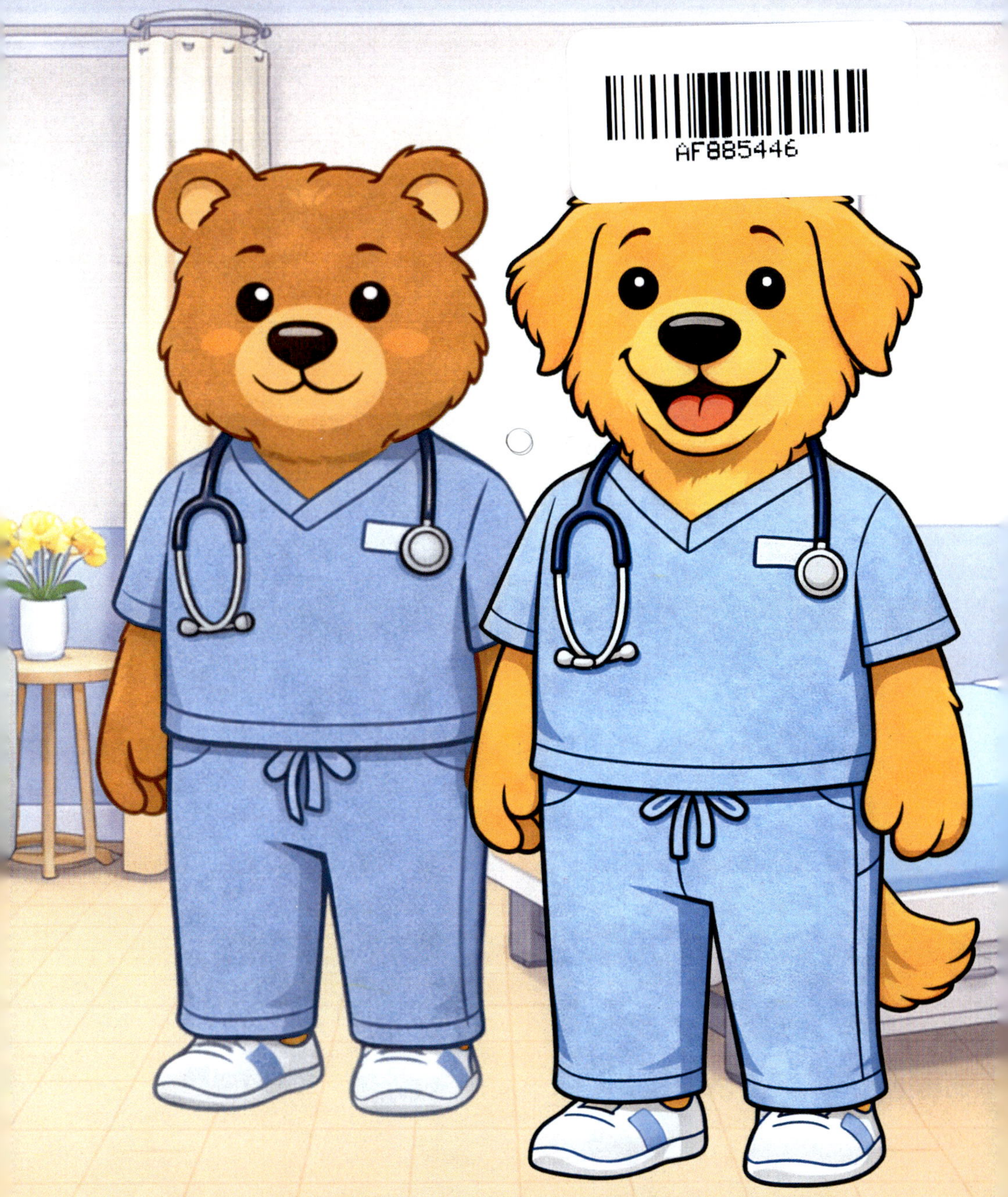

Nurses are kind, caring, and
help people feel better.

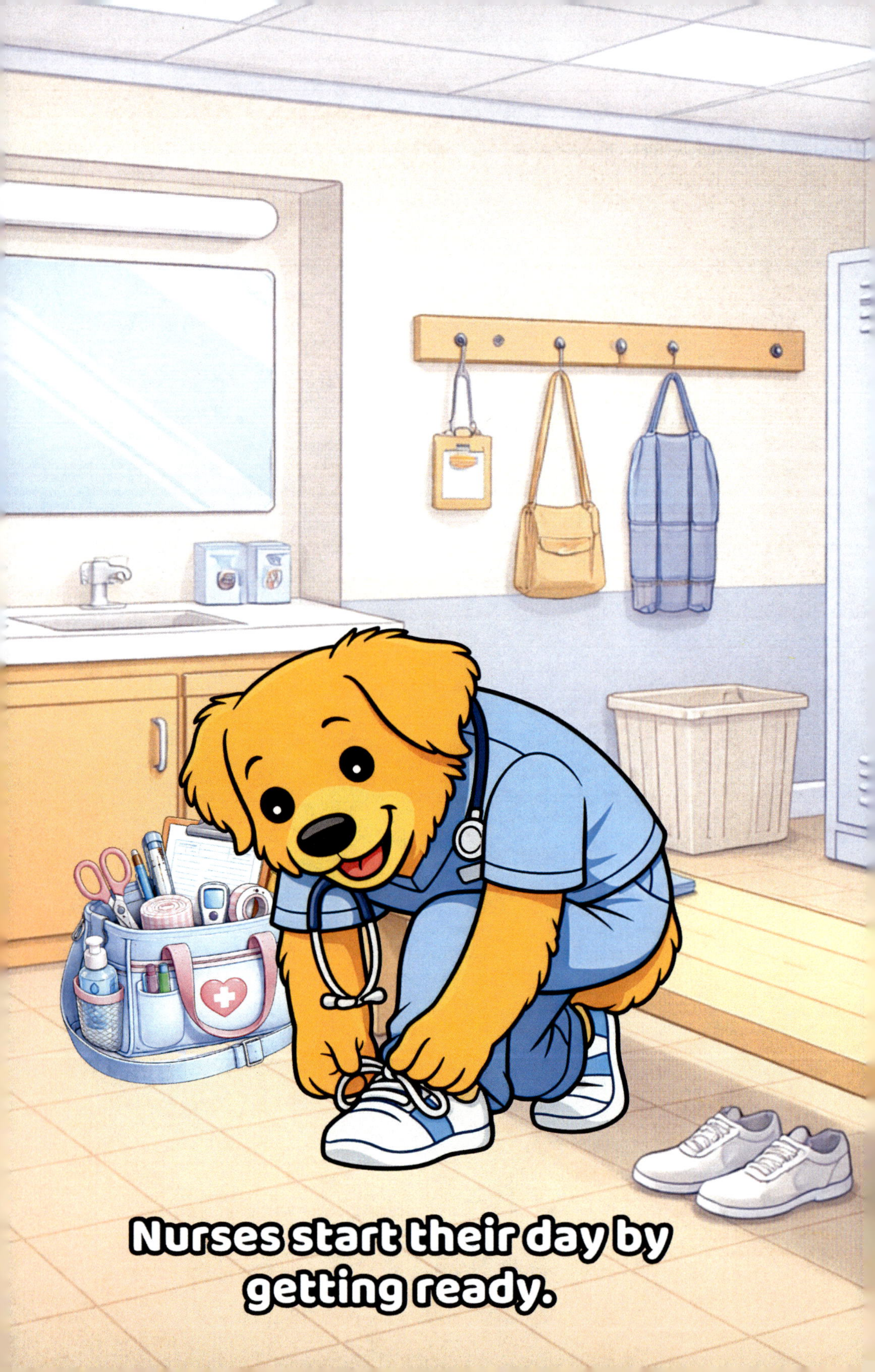

Nurses start their day by getting ready.

They put on their scrubs and gather their tools.

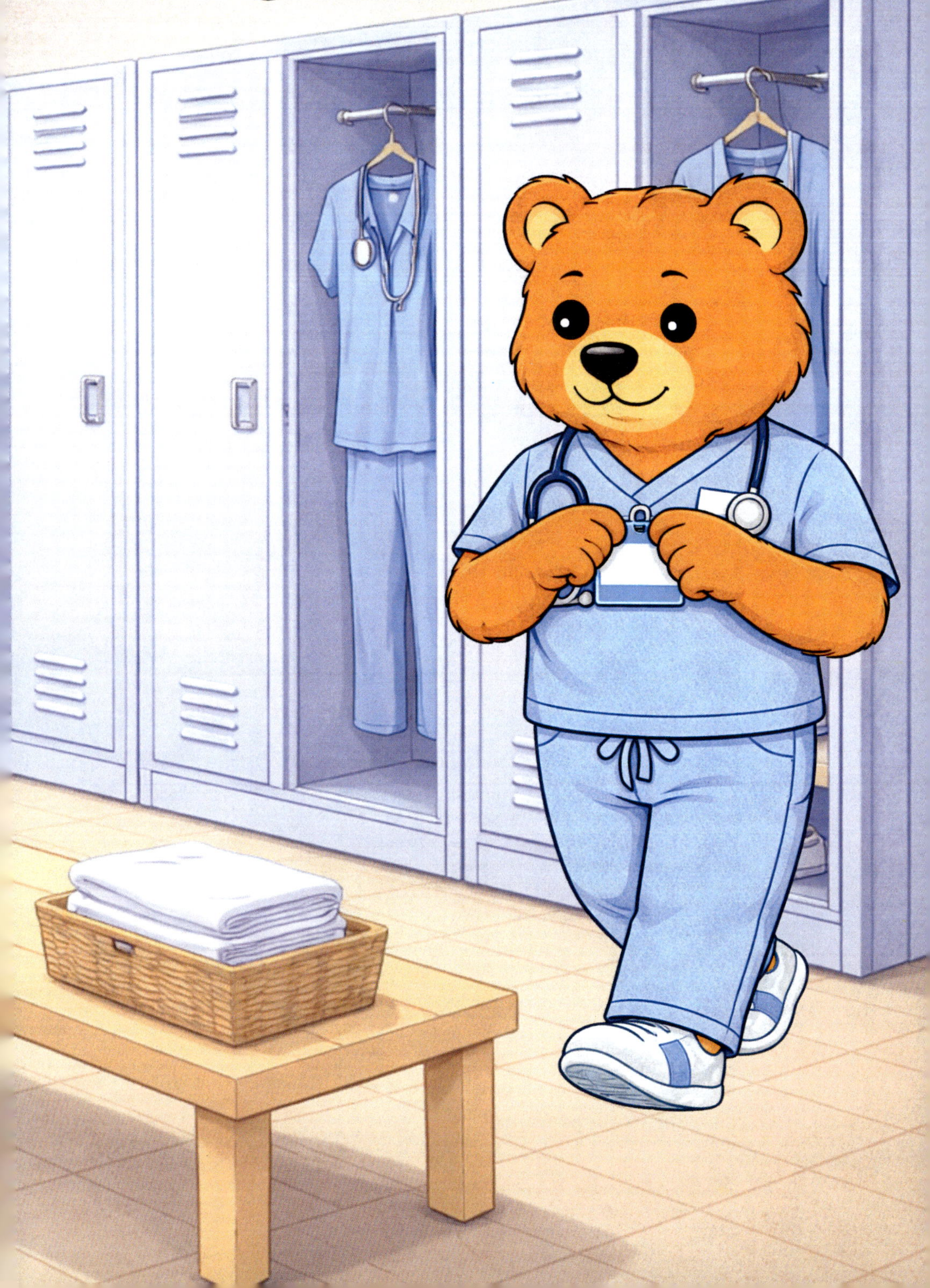

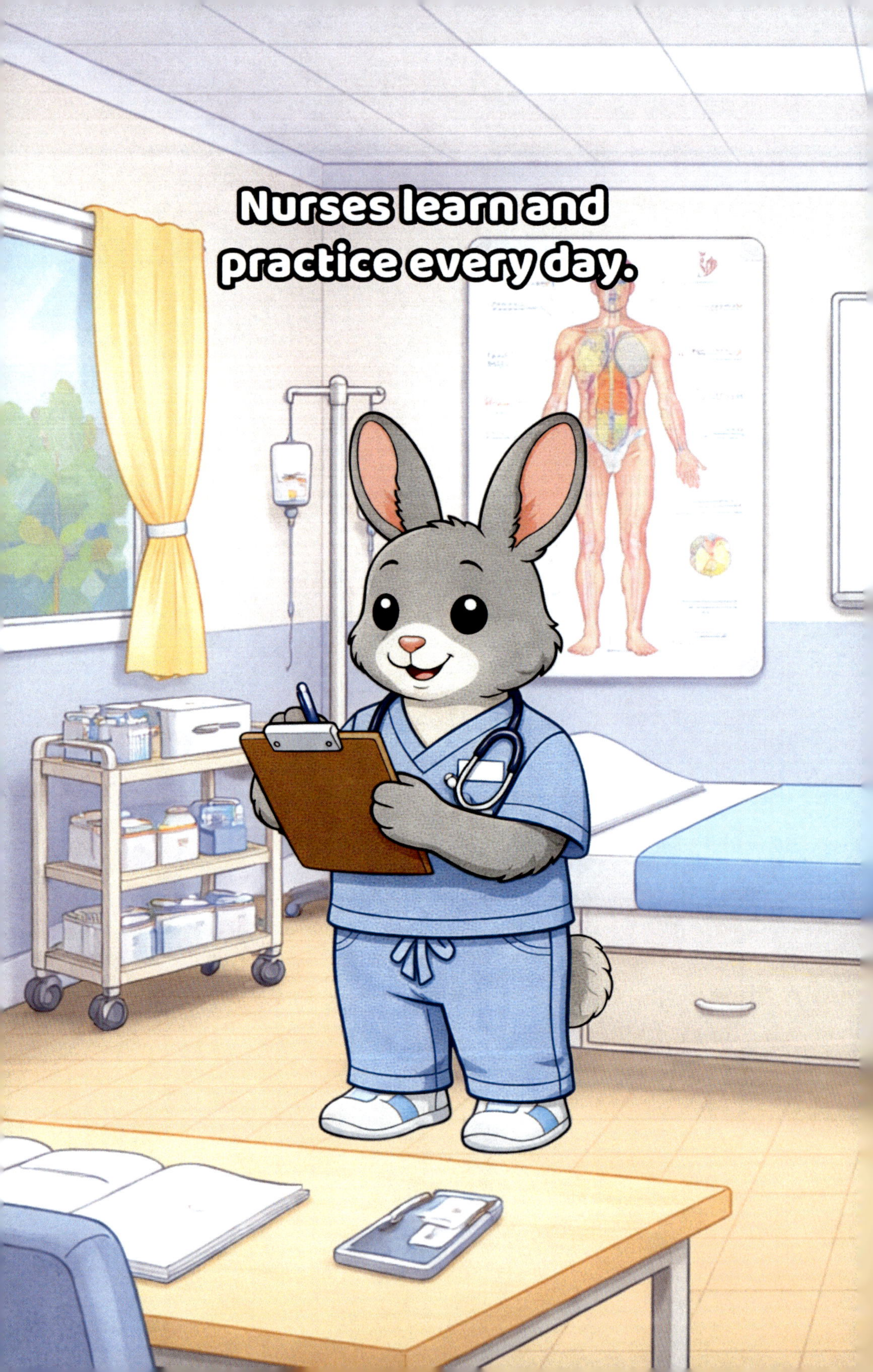

Nurses learn and practice every day.

This helps them take the best care of others.

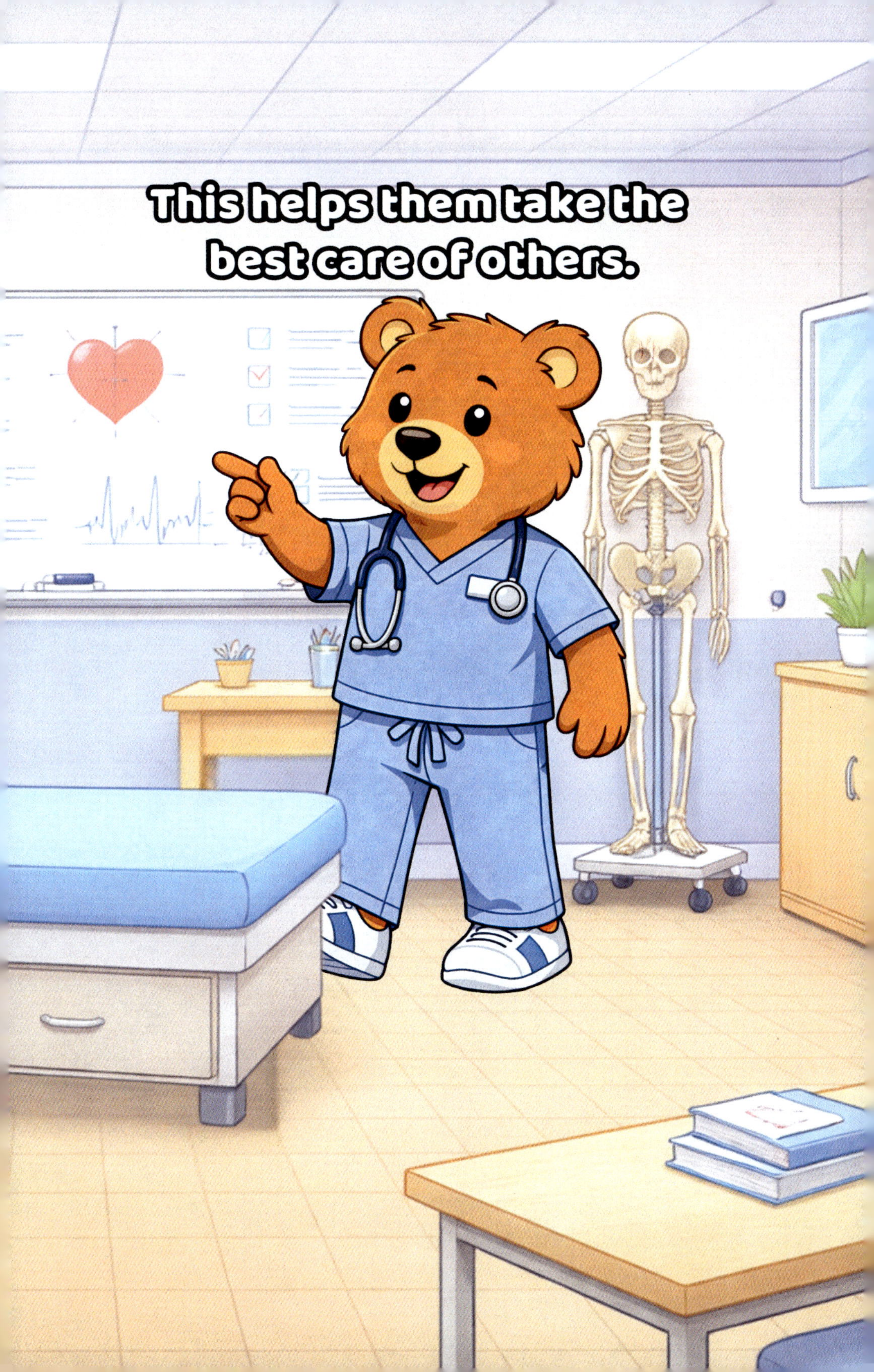

Nursing is all about teamwork.

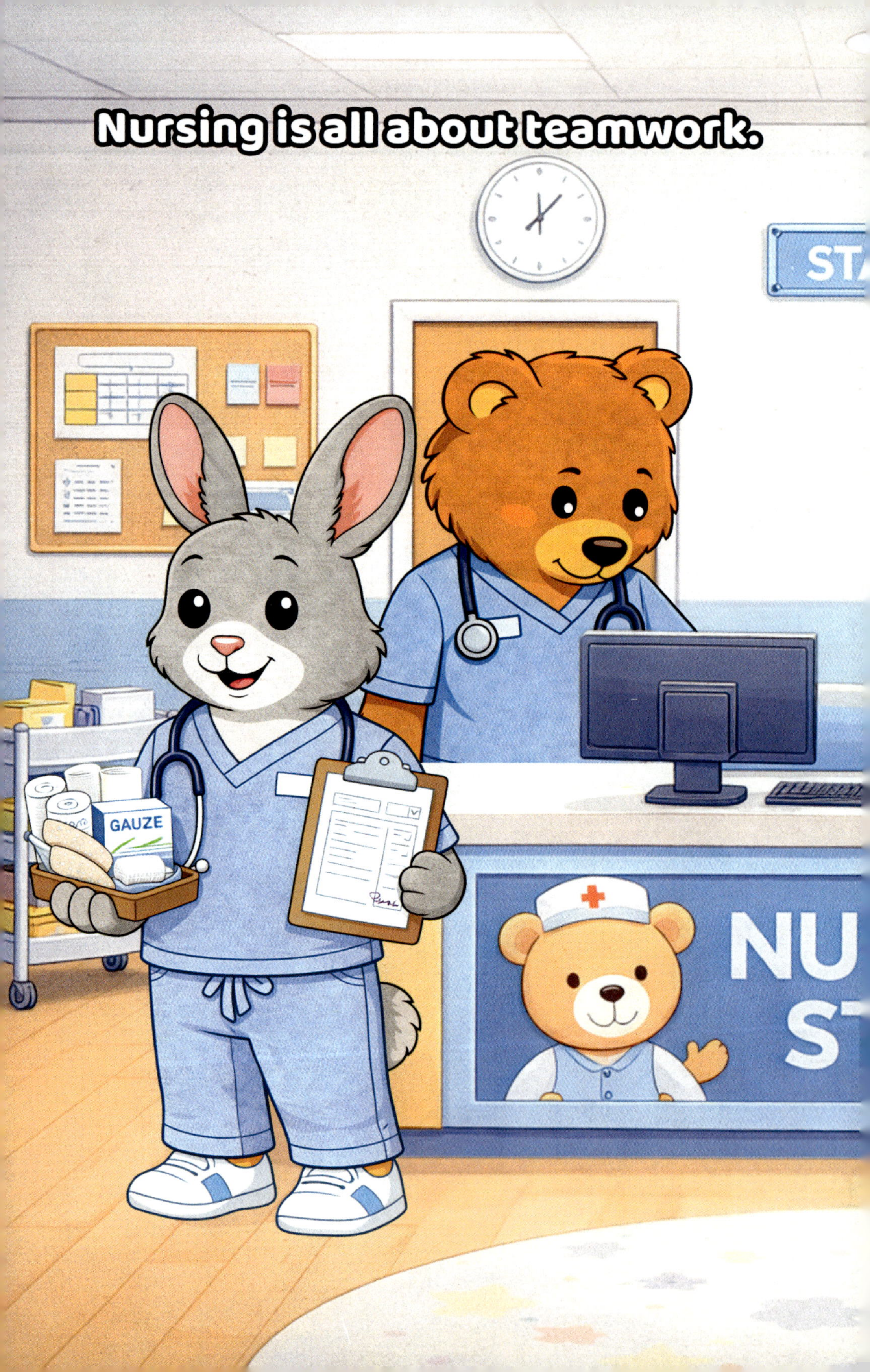

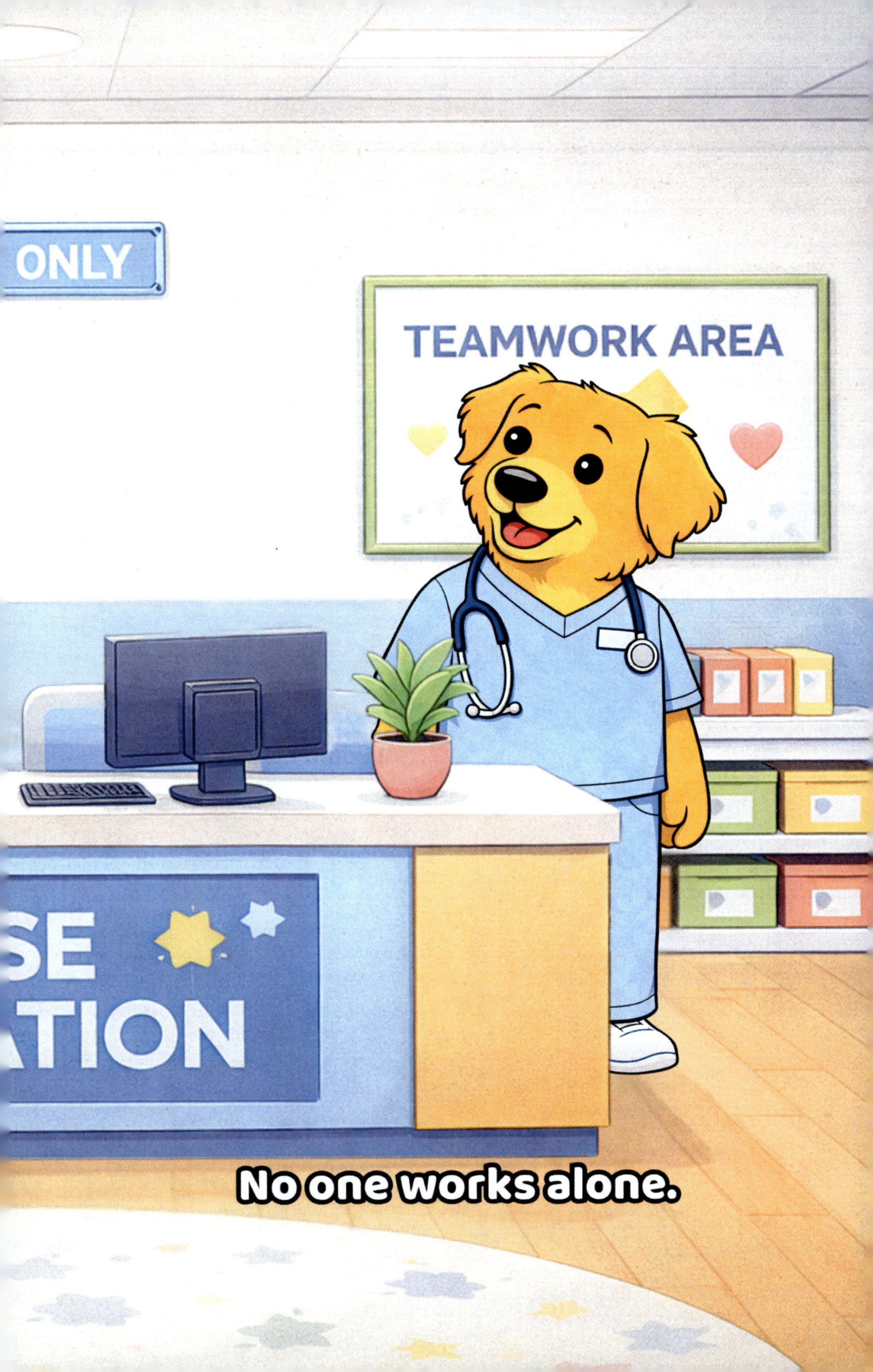

No one works alone.

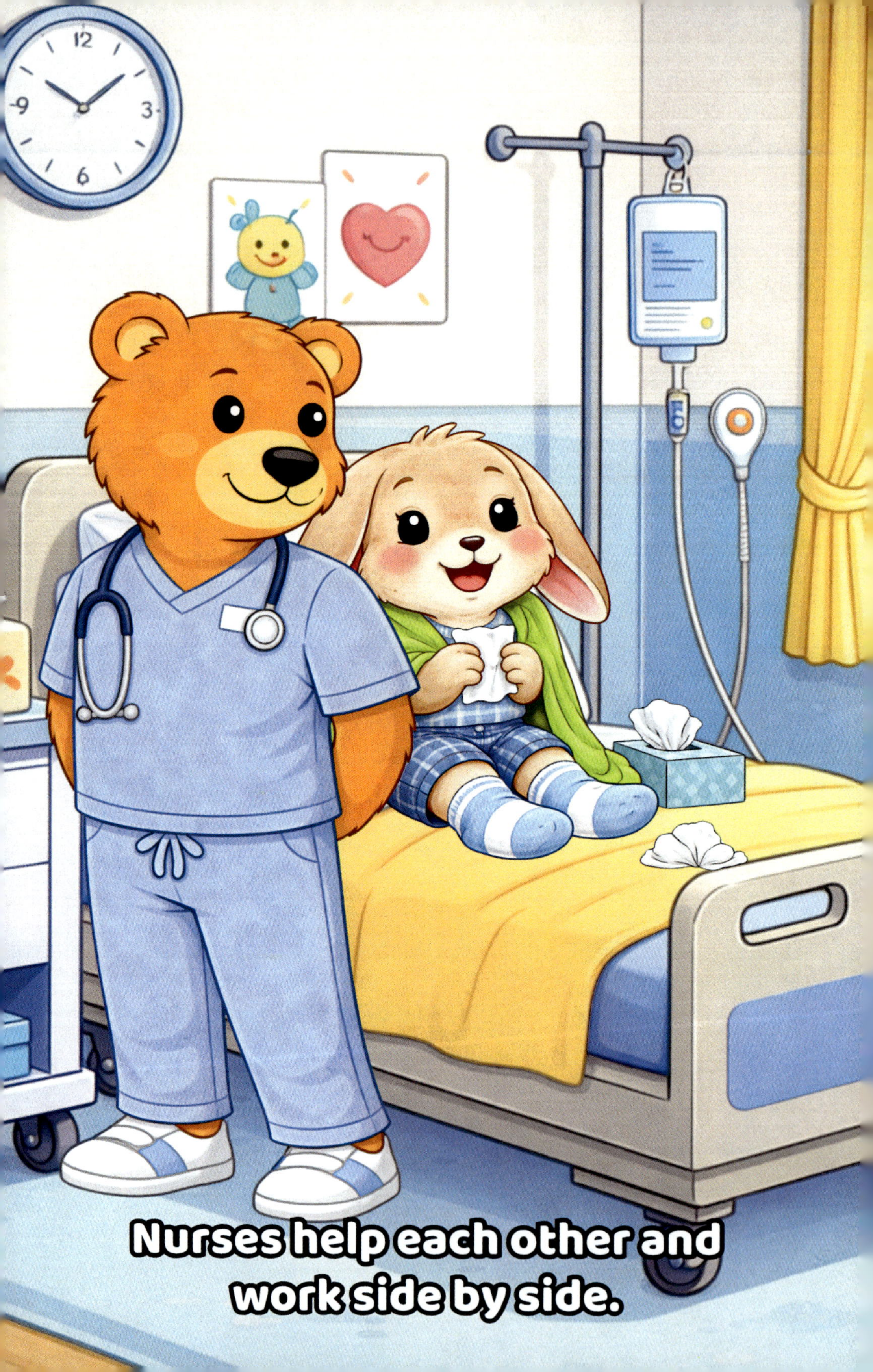

Nurses help each other and
work side by side.

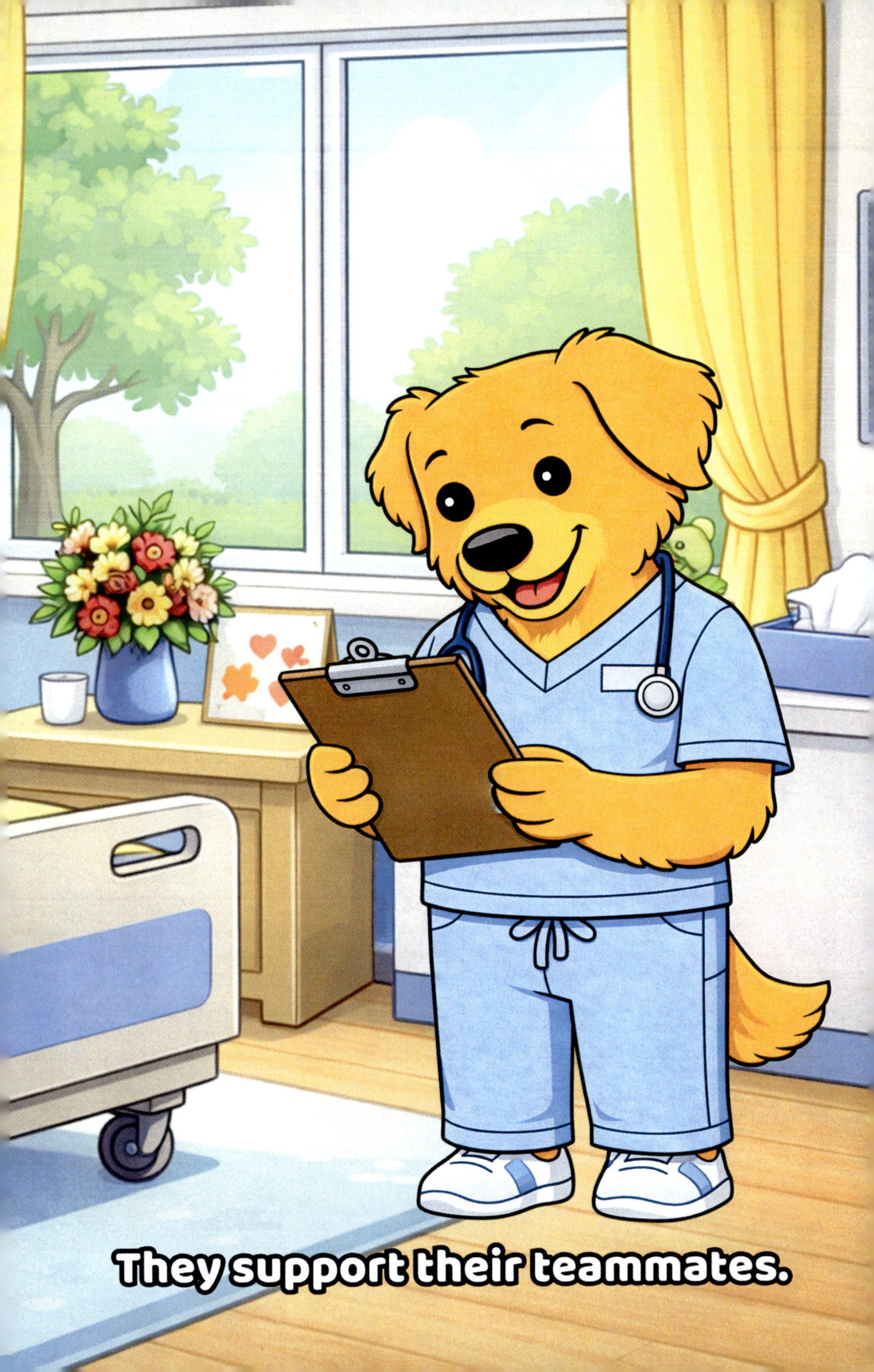

They support their teammates.

Nurses check how people are feeling.

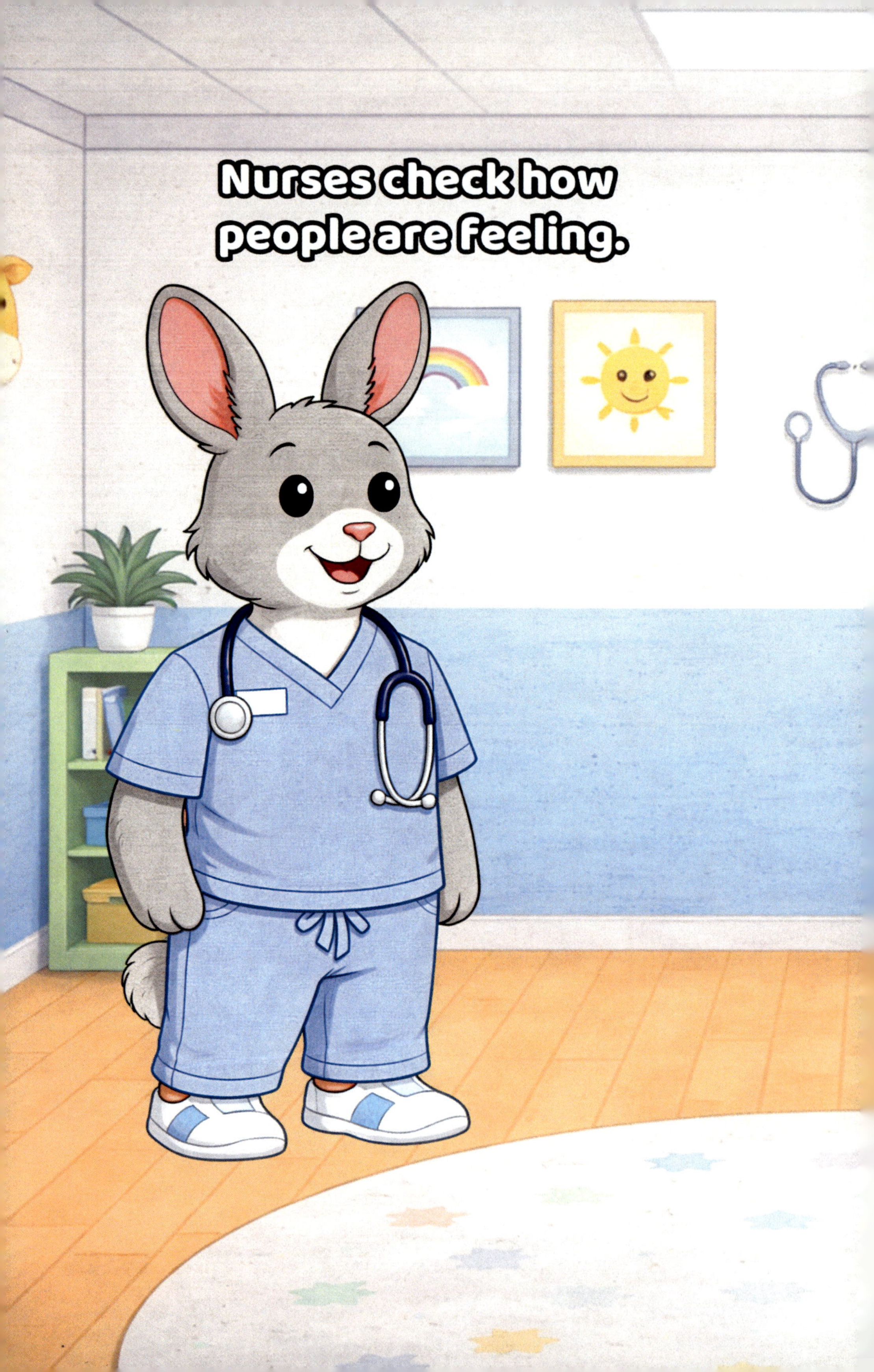

They listen, look, and make sure everything is okay.

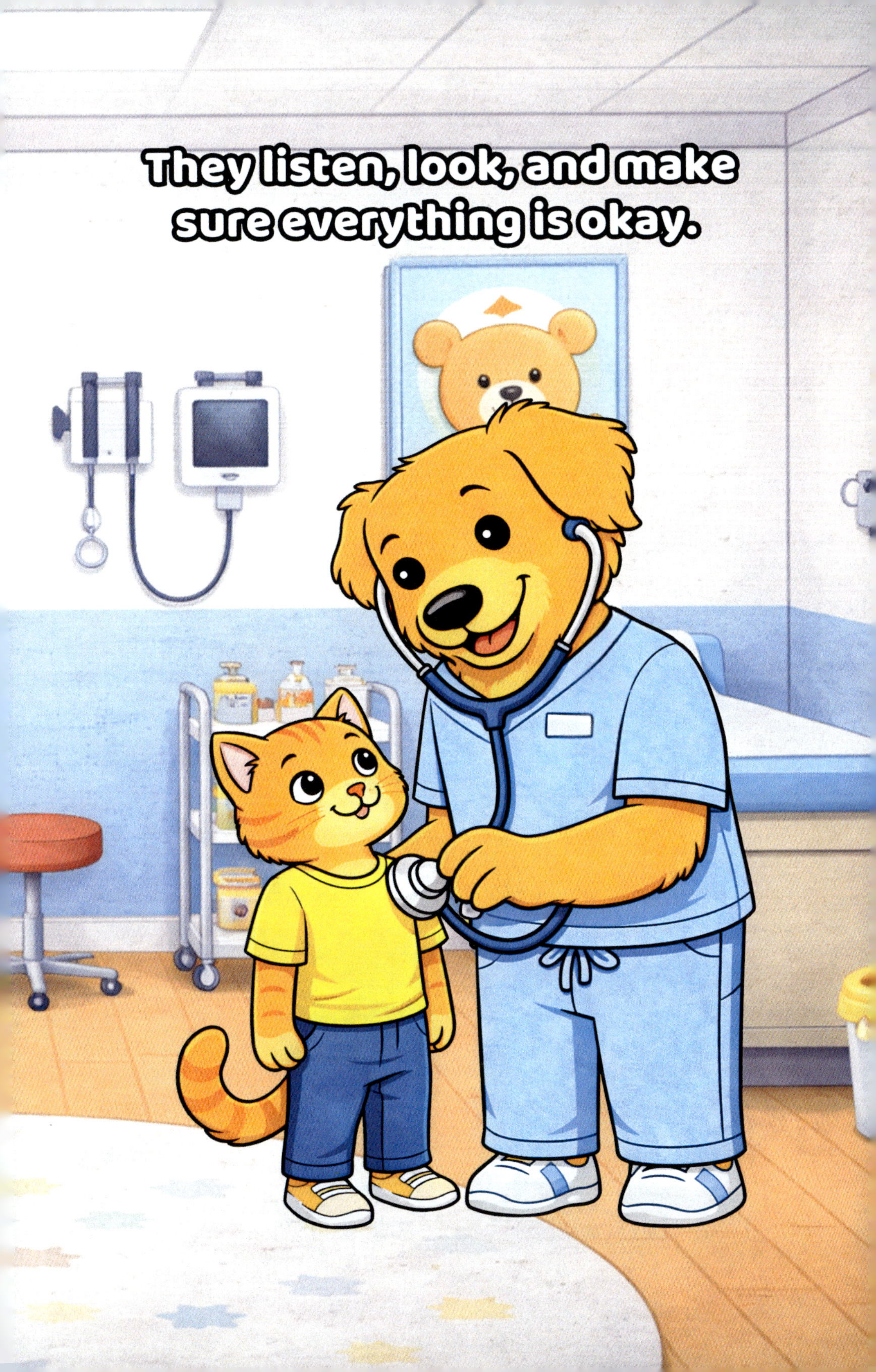

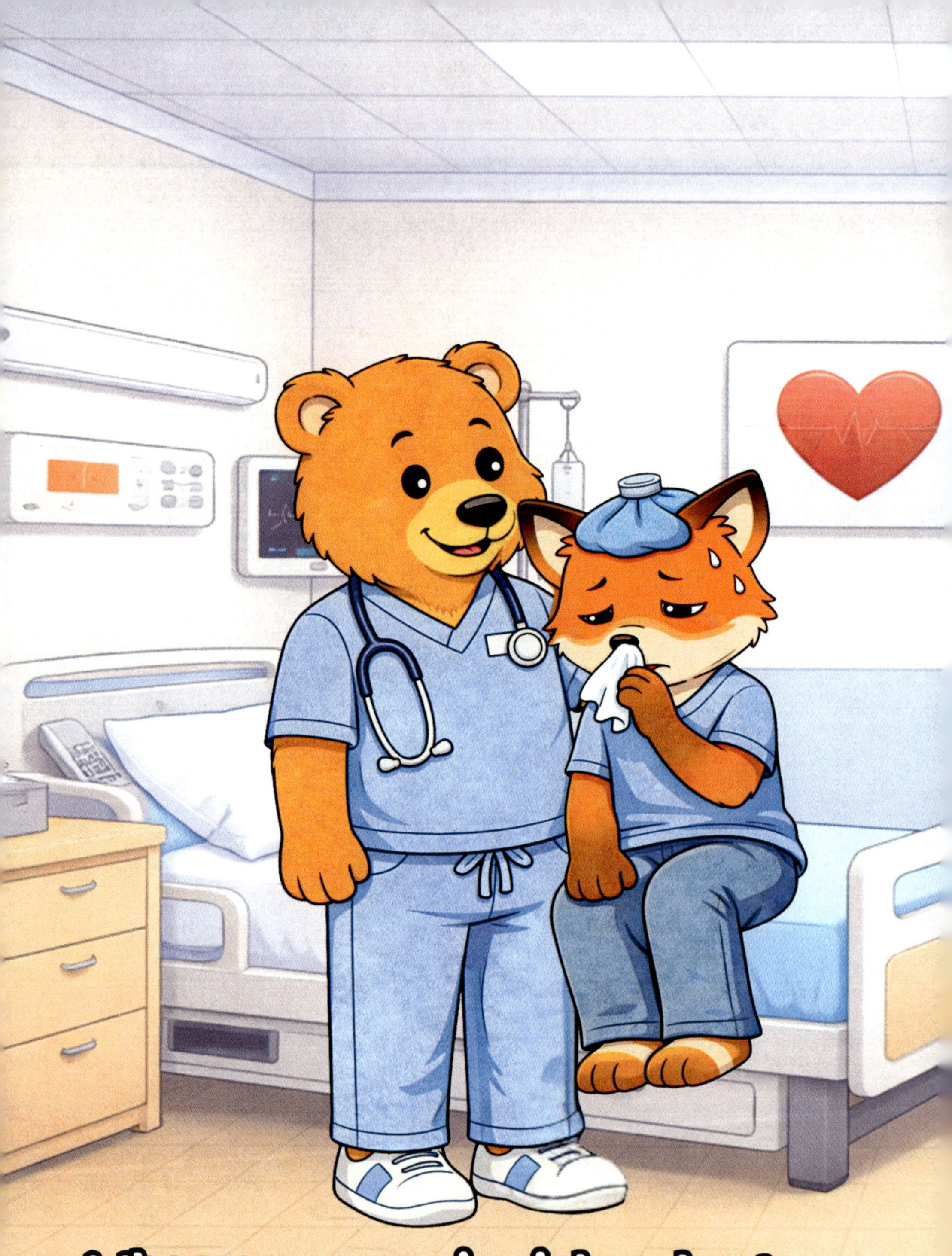

When someone is sick or hurt,
nurses help them.

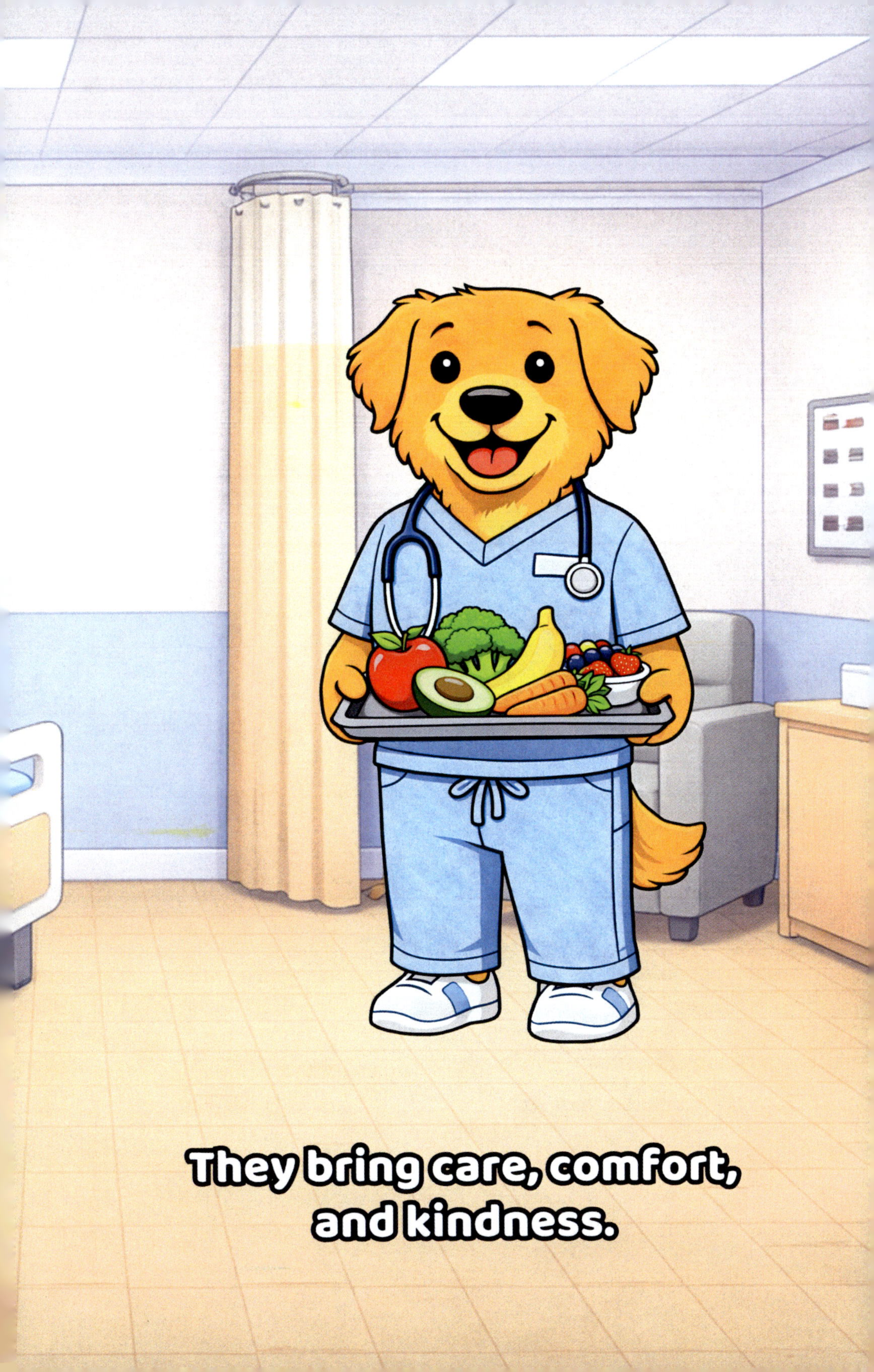

They bring care, comfort,
and kindness.

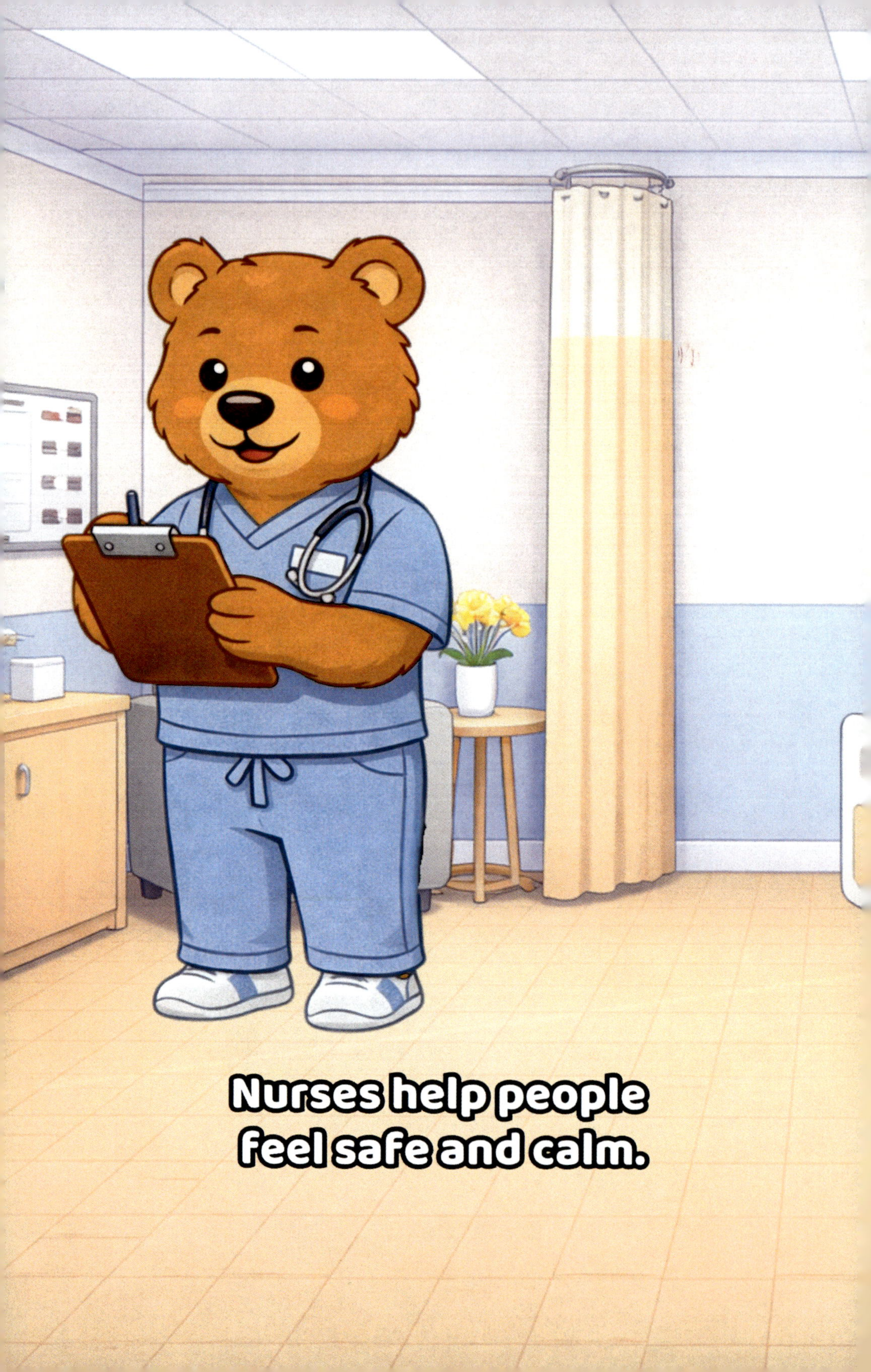

Nurses help people
feel safe and calm.

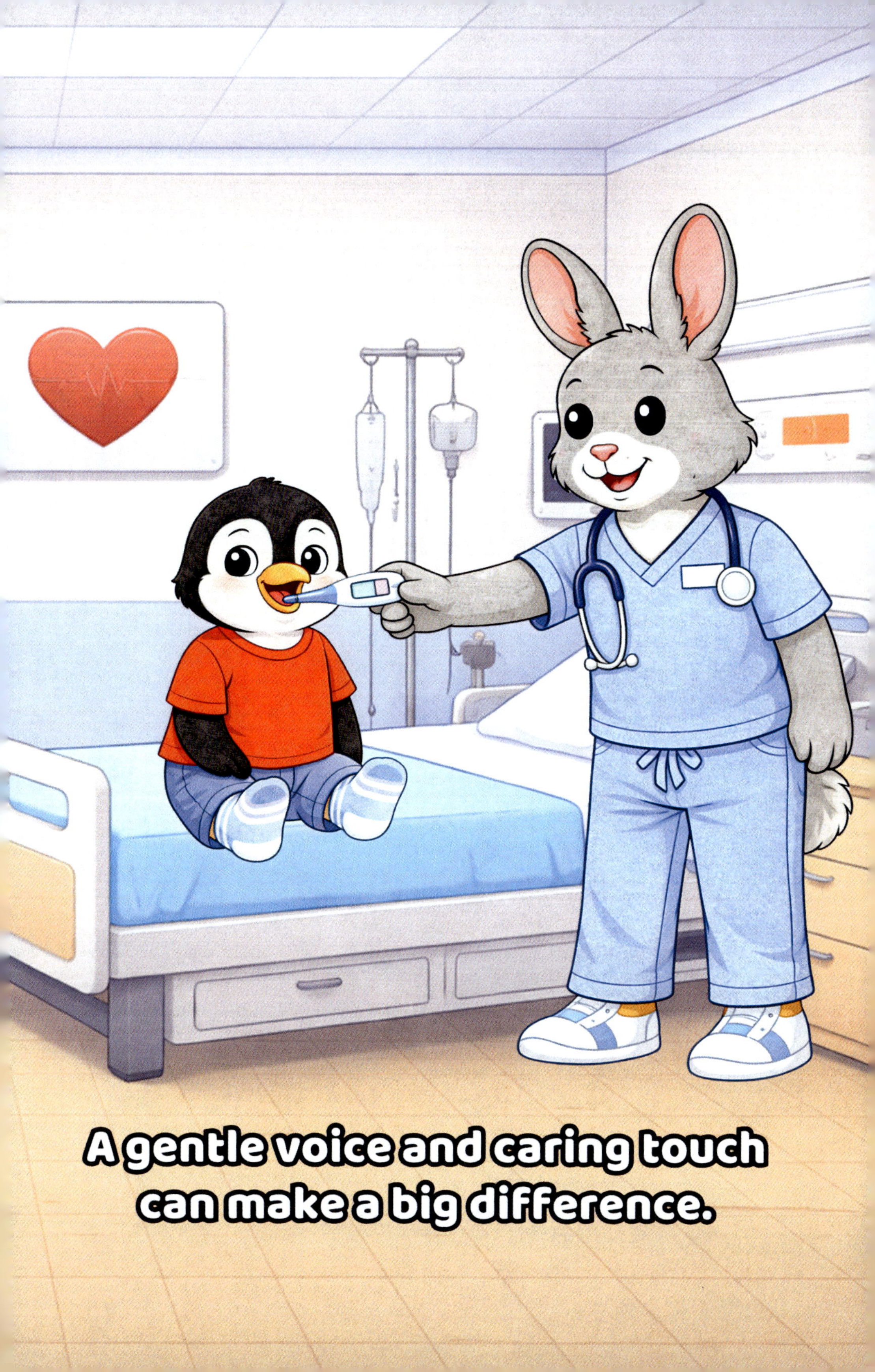

A gentle voice and caring touch
can make a big difference.

Nurses work in many places.

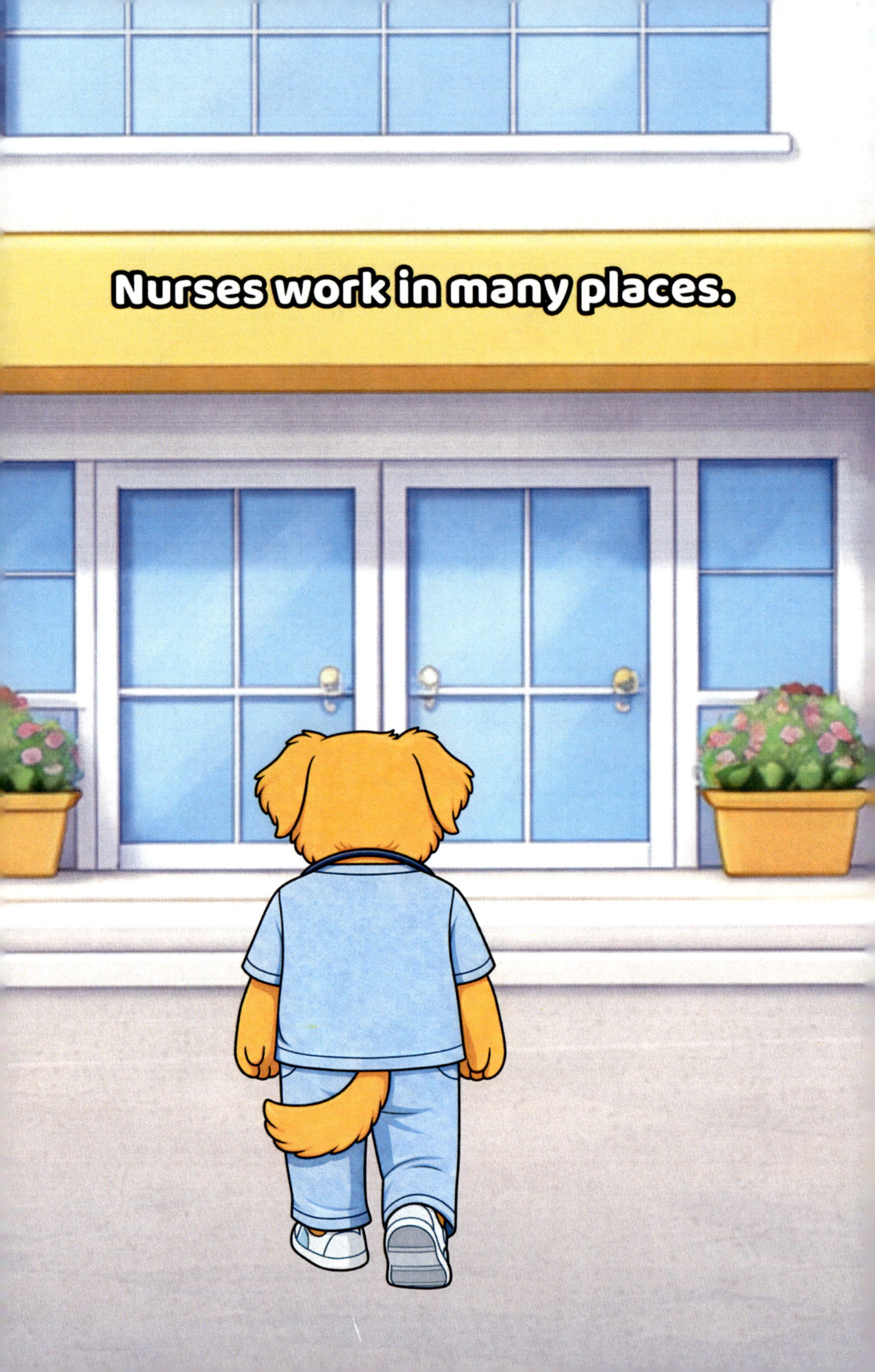

Hospitals, clinics, and beyond.

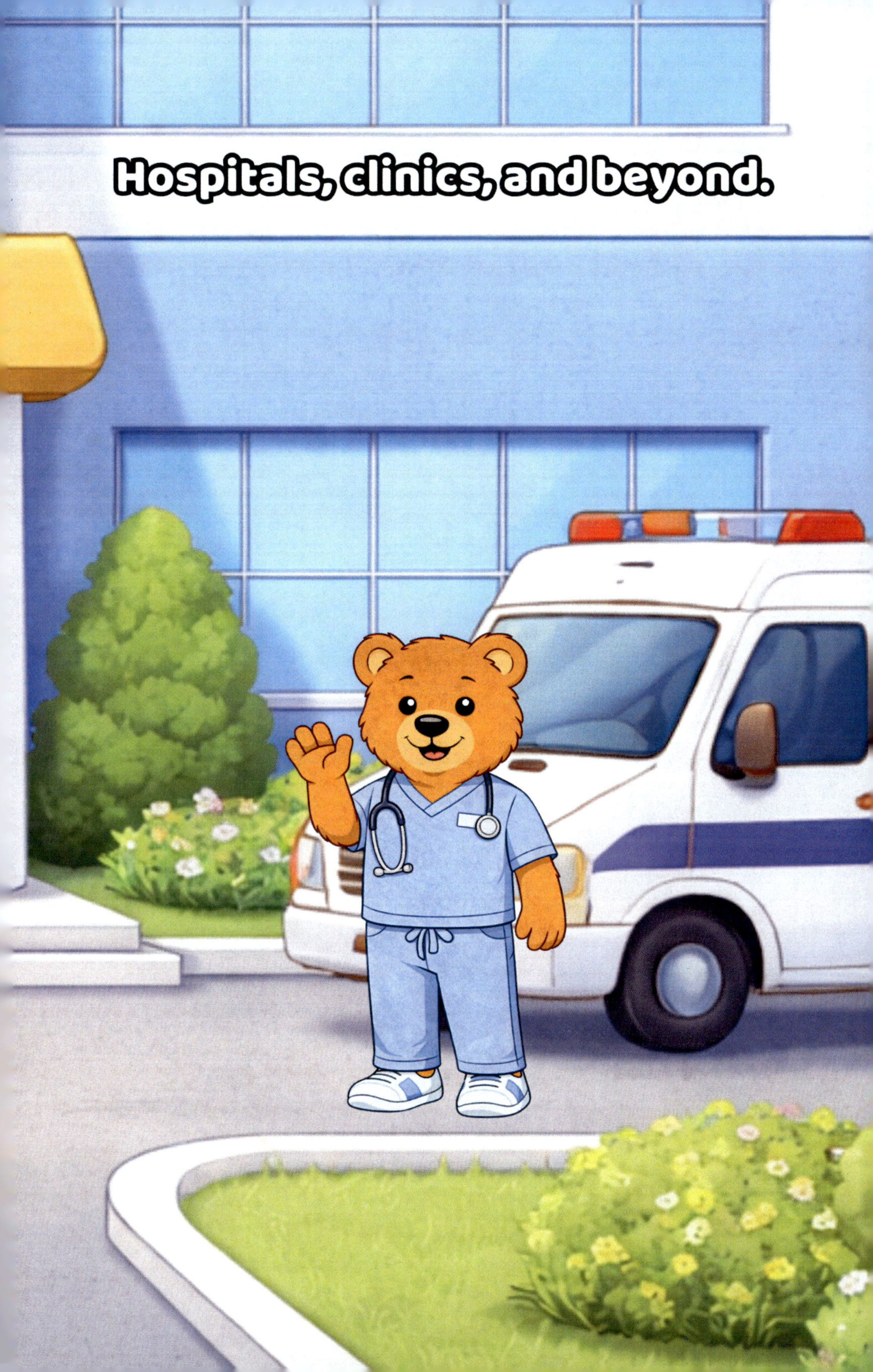

Nurses care for
more than just patients.

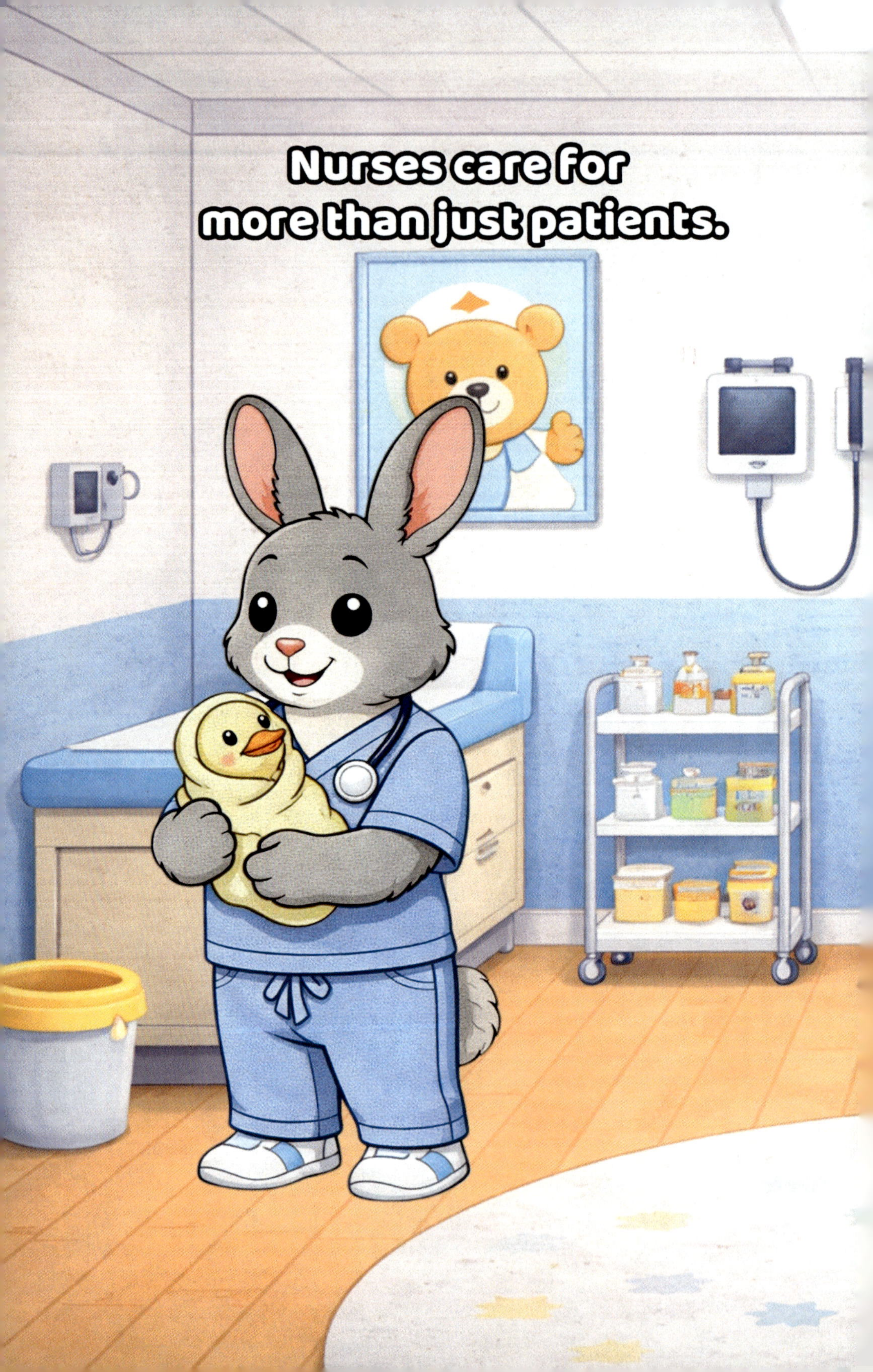

They help families feel better too.

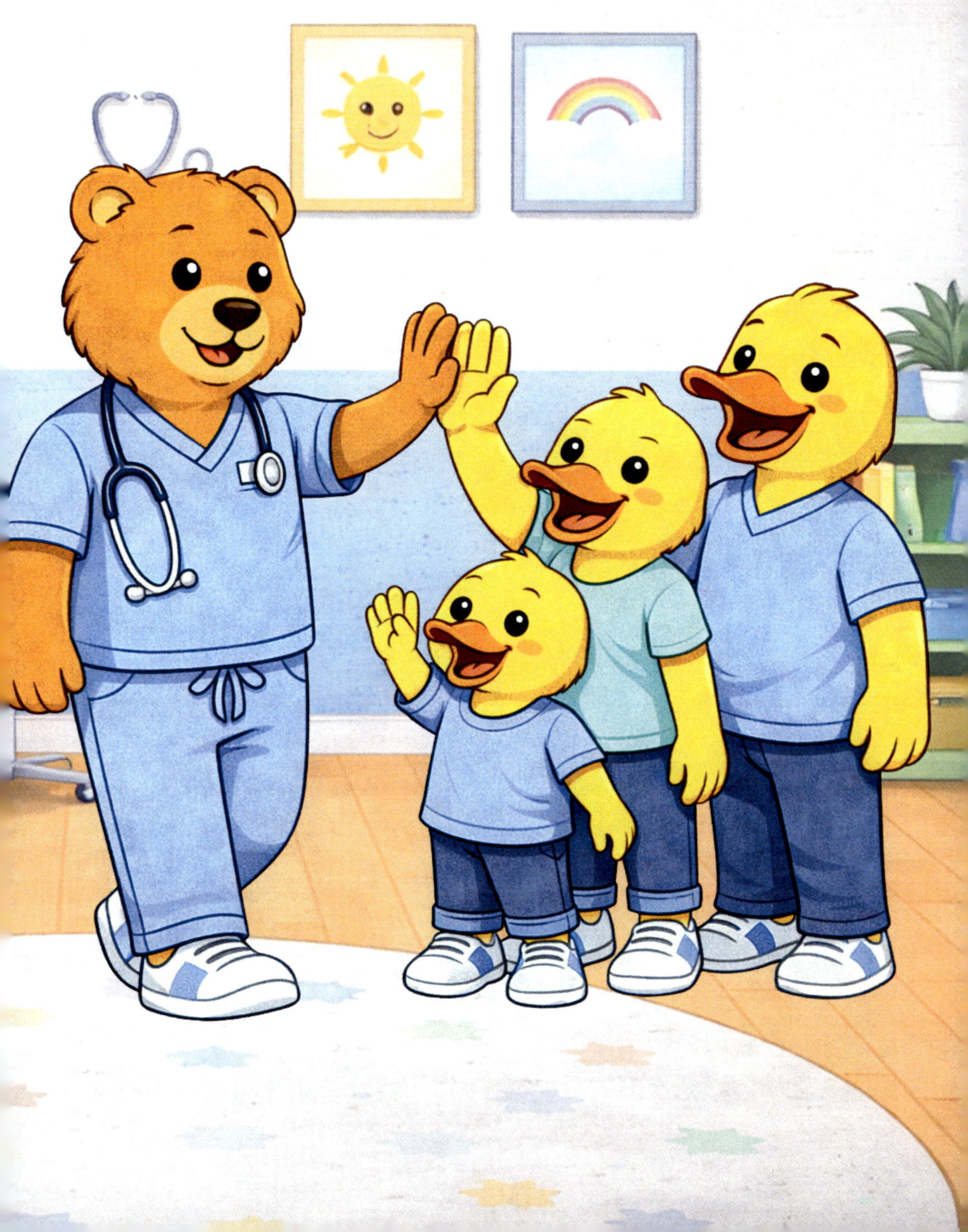

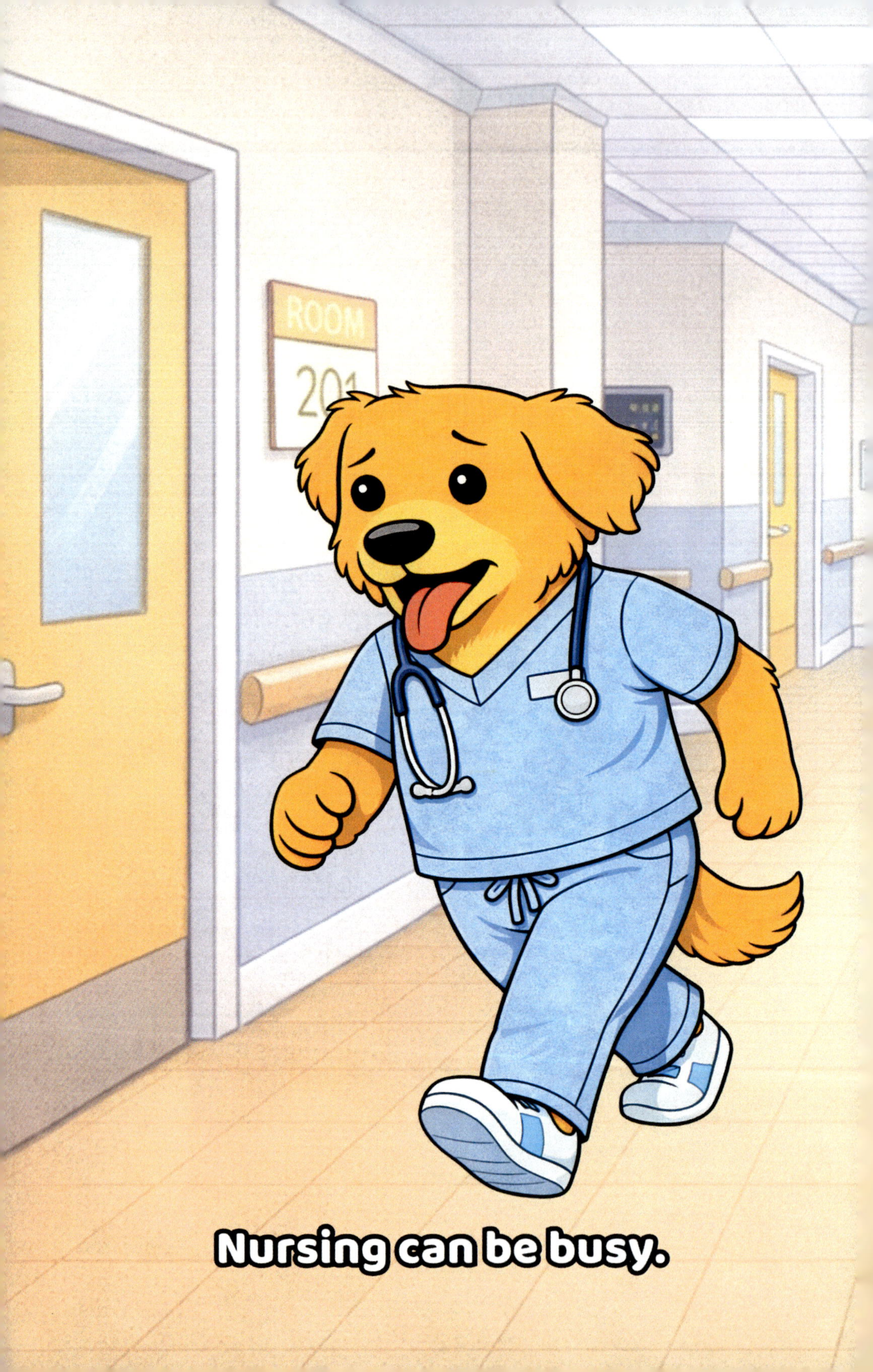

Nursing can be busy.

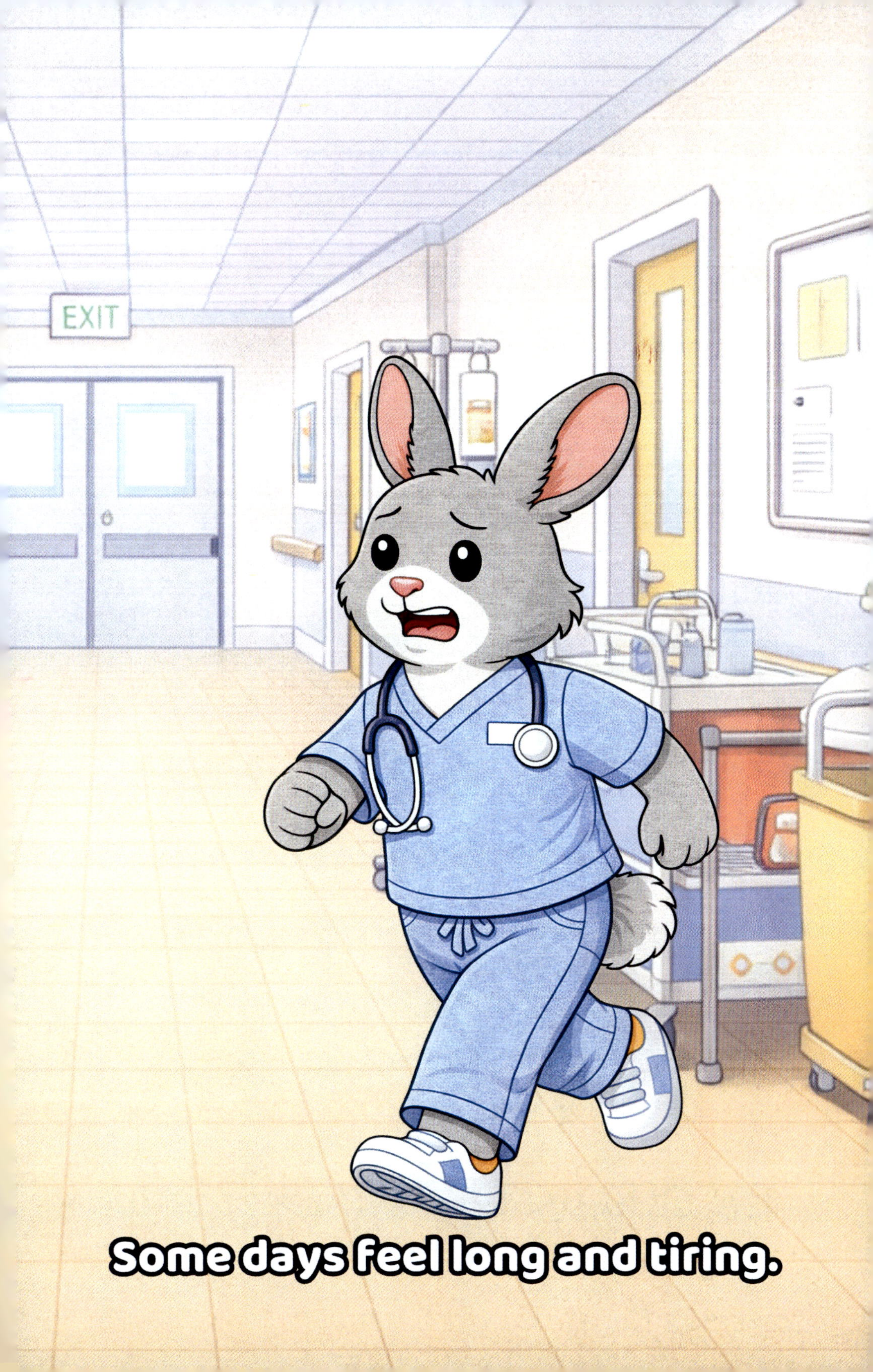

Some days feel long and tiring.

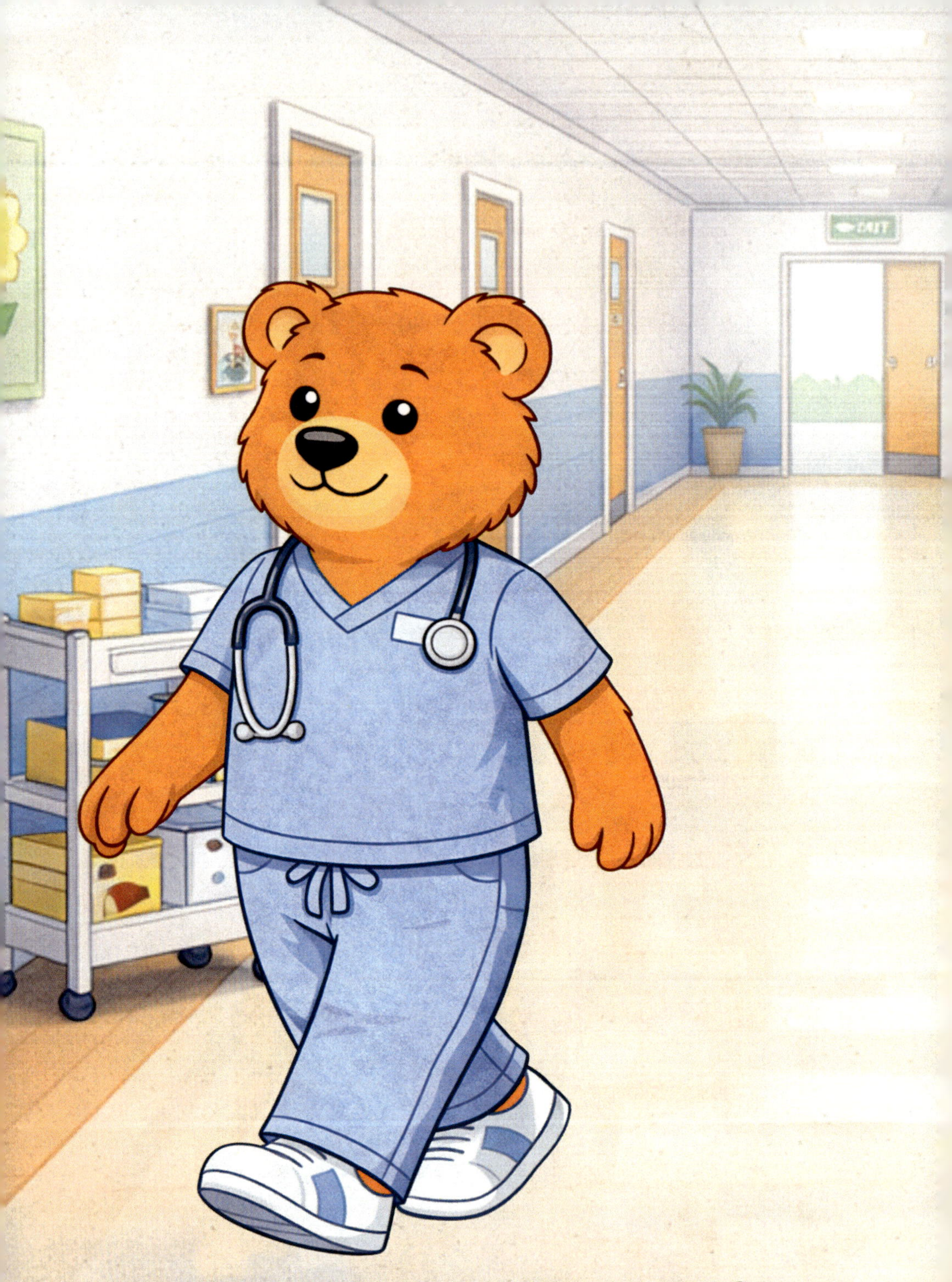

Even then, nurses keep going
and do their best.

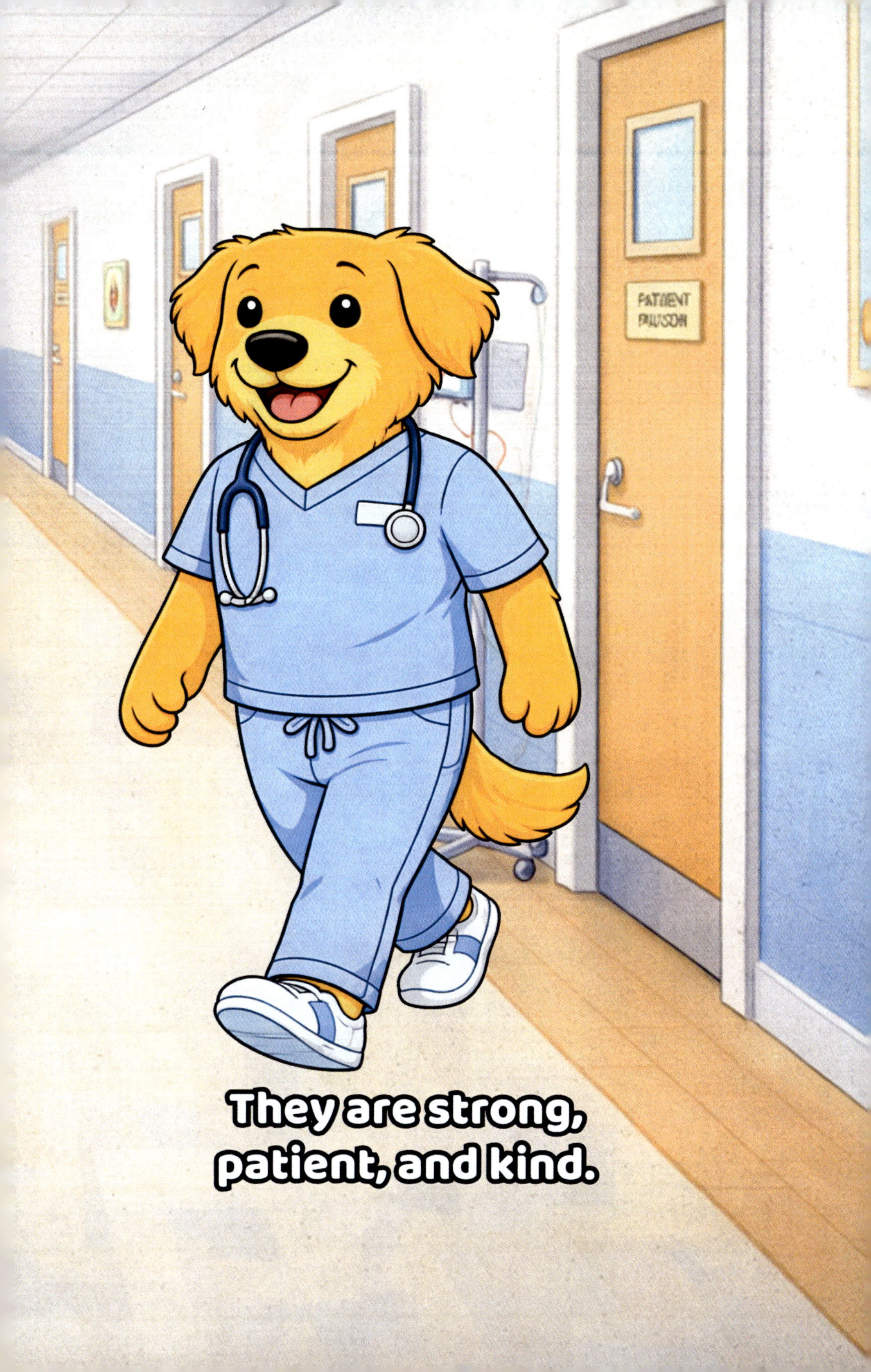

They are strong,
patient, and kind.

Nurses matter.

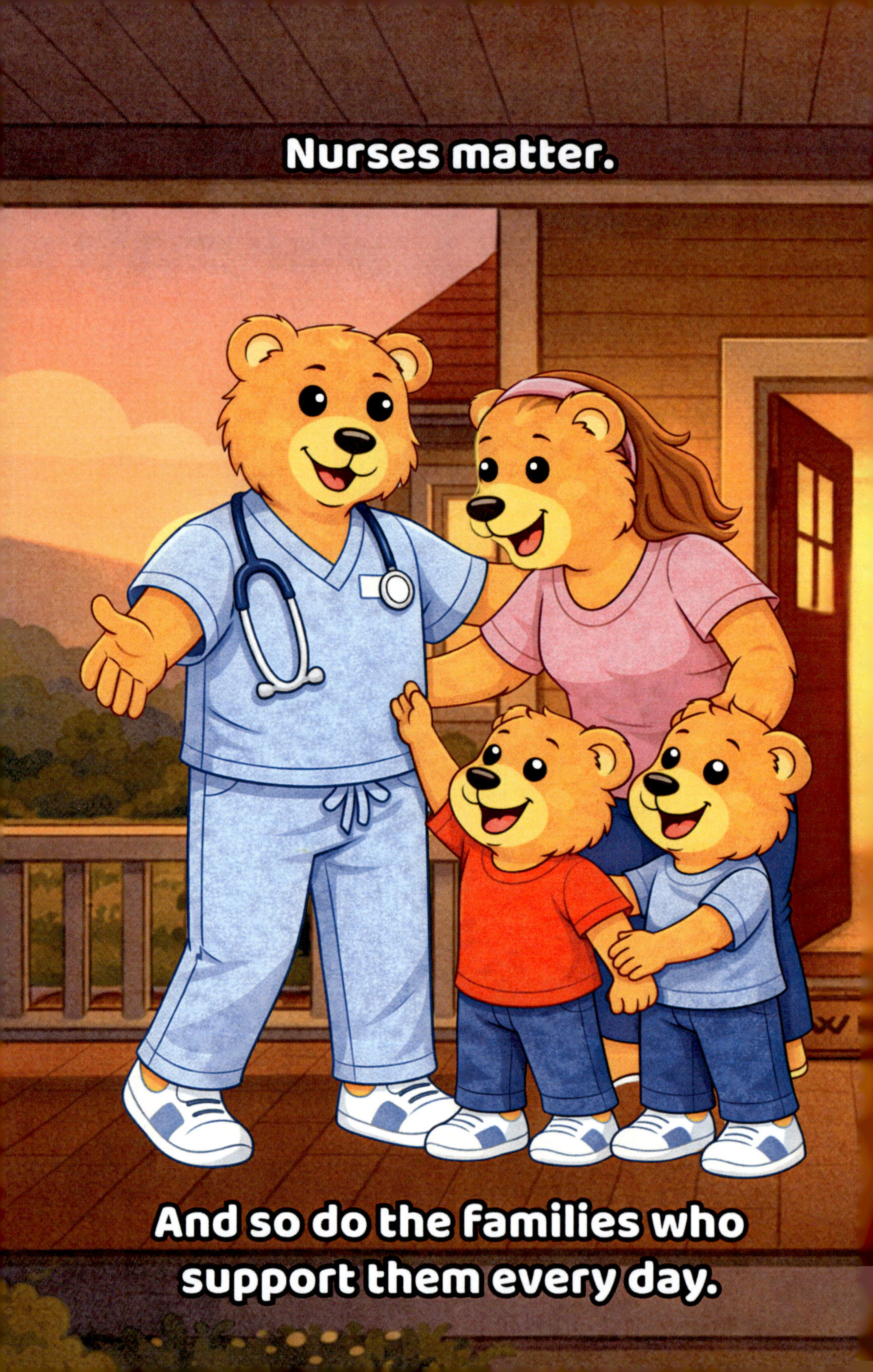

And so do the families who
support them every day.

Made in United States
North Haven, CT
05 November 2026

21765506R60015